PREGNANCY WITH TYPE 1 OR TYPE 2 DIABETES

(A real-life guide)

Dr. Macklene. C. Jones

INTRODUCTION

1

WHAT EXACTLY IS DIABETES?
DIABETES TYPES DURING PREGNANCY
THE IMPACT OF DIABETES ON PREGNANCY

2

PRECONCEPTION PLANNING
THE SIGNIFICANCE OF PRECONCEPTION PLANNING
COUNSELING BEFORE CONCEPTION
MEDICATION ADMINISTRATION

3

PREGNANCY BLOOD SUGAR CONTROL DURING PREGNANCY
MONITORING BLOOD SUGAR LEVELS
WHAT EXACTLY IS SMBG?
HOW TO CARRY OUT SMBG
WHEN SHOULD BLOOD SUGAR LEVELS BE CHECKED?
TARGET BLOOD SUGAR LEVELS DURING PREGNANCY
KEEPING TRACK OF YOUR BLOOD SUGAR LEVELS
WHAT EXACTLY IS CGM?
HOW DOES CGM FUNCTION?
CGM ADVANTAGES DURING PREGNANCY
CGM ALLOWS YOU TO CONTROL YOUR BLOOD SUGAR LEVELS
CGM RESTRICTIONS
WHAT REALLY IS HbA1c?
WHAT ROLE DOES HbA1c PLAY IN BLOOD SUGAR CONTROL?
WHEN IS HbA1c TESTING PERFORMED DURING PREGNANCY?
HbA1c VALUES TO AIM FOR DURING PREGNANCY
HbA1c LIMITATIONS
FACTORS INFLUENCING BLOOD SUGAR LEVELS DURING PREGNANCY INCLUDE HORMONAL CHANGES
INSULIN SENSITIVITY
DIETARY AND NUTRITIONAL REQUIREMENTS
PHYSICAL EXERCISE AND ACTIVITIES
SIGNIFICANT FACTORS TO CONSIDER WHEN IT COMES TO PHYSICAL ACTIVITY AND EXERCISE DURING PREGNANCY
ILLNESS AND STRESS
THE SIGNIFICANCE OF BLOOD SUGAR MONITORING DURING PREGNANCY: THE DANGERS OF UNCONTROLLED BLOOD SUGAR LEVELS DURING PREGNANCY
ADVANTAGES OF KEEPING TARGET BLOOD SUGAR LEVELS DURING PREGNANCY
THE ROLE OF HEALTHCARE PROFESSIONALS IN PREGNANCY BLOOD SUGAR MONITORING
WORKING WITH A HEALTHCARE TEAM; TIPS FOR SUCCESSFUL BLOOD SUGAR MONITORING DURING PREGNANCY

MAINTAINING A RECORD OF BLOOD SUGAR LEVELS
DETECTING TRENDS AND MODIFYING TREATMENT
TREATMENT PLAN OR DRUG REGIMEN
ADDRESSING CONCERNS AND DIFFICULTIES
INSULIN THERAPY
TYPES OF INSULIN
MEAL PLANNING AND NUTRITION
EXERCISE DURING PREGNANCY

4

PROBABLE COMPLICATIONS OF DIABETES IN PREGNANCY

5

FETAL MONITORING
CLASSIFICATION OF FETAL ULTRASOUNDS
WHEN PERFORMING FETAL ULTRASOUNDS
BENEFITS OF FETAL ULTRASOUNDS
LIMITATIONS OF FETAL ULTRASOUNDS
OVERVIEW OF VARIOUS FETAL MONITORING TECHNIQUES
TYPES OF ULTRASOUND SCANS
HOW ULTRASOUND WORKS
TYPES OF ULTRASOUNDS USED FOR FETAL MONITORING
HOW ULTRASOUNDS MIGHT DETECT DIABETIC PROBLEMS DURING PREGNANCY
HOW TO FEEL HEART RATE MONITORING DURING FETAL LIFE
FETAL HEART RATE MONITORING METHODOLOGY
WHEN IS FETAL HEART RATE MONITORING COMMONLY UTILIZED DURING PREGNANCY?
WHAT FETAL HEART RATE MONITORING MIGHT REVEAL DIABETIC PROBLEMS DURING PREGNANCY?
WHAT EXACTLY IS A NON-STRESS TEST (NST)?
HOW THE NON-STRESS TEST IS CARRIED OUT
HOW A NON-STRESS TEST CAN DETECT DIABETES PROBLEMS IN PREGNANCY
A BIOPHYSICAL PROFILE (BPP)
HOW IS A BIOPHYSICAL PROFILE PERFORMED?
HOW CAN A BIOPHYSICAL PROFILE DETECT DIABETIC ISSUES DURING PREGNANCY?
CONTRACTION STRESS TEST (CST)
HOW THE CONTRACTION STRESS TEST IS CARRIED OUT
WHAT DOES THE CONTRACTION STRESS TEST SHOW?
HOW A CONTRACTION STRESS TEST MIGHT REVEAL DIABETIC PROBLEMS IN PREGNANCY
COLLABORATION BETWEEN HEALTHCARE PRACTITIONERS AND PATIENTS

6

LABOR AND DELIVERY
LABOR INDUCTION

Mode of Distribution
Postnatal Care
Breastfeeding With Diabetes

<u>7</u>

Postpartum Care
Breastfeeding and Medications
Follow-up Treatment
Options for Contraception

<u>8</u>

Long-Term Health Consequences
Diabetes Management Following Pregnancy
Preparing For a Future Pregnancy
Considerations for Emotional and Mental Health

<u>CONCLUSION</u>

Introduction

Diabetes is a chronic metabolic condition marked by elevated blood glucose or sugar levels. Diabetes is a primary source of morbidity and mortality for millions of individuals globally. Diabetes can have major consequences for women during pregnancy, harming both the mother and the growing fetus. Diabetes-complicated pregnancies necessitate meticulous management to provide the best possible outcome for both mother and child.

This book is a complete reference to diabetes management throughout pregnancy, covering topics such as preconception planning, blood sugar control, fetal monitoring, delivery, postpartum care, and long-term maintenance. The book is aimed at healthcare providers who work with diabetic women, as well as diabetic women who are planning or are currently pregnant.

The first chapter discusses diabetes in general, including the numerous forms of diabetes and their causes, symptoms, and treatment choices. The chapter also goes into the effects of diabetes on pregnancy and the potential issues that can occur.

The second chapter focuses on preconception planning, which is critical for diabetic women who want to become pregnant. Preconception counseling, blood sugar control before pregnancy, medication management, and other considerations to consider before getting pregnant are all covered in this chapter.

The third chapter goes into insulin therapy, which is an important part of diabetes control during pregnancy. The chapter discusses insulin types, insulin delivery techniques, and how to modify insulin doses in response to changing blood sugar levels.

The fourth chapter delves into the potential consequences of diabetes during pregnancy, such as gestational diabetes, pre-eclampsia, and fetal distress syndrome. The chapter also goes into how to diagnose and handle these issues.

The fifth chapter focuses on fetal monitoring, which is crucial for safeguarding the developing fetus's health and well-being. The chapter discusses fetal monitoring techniques, including ultrasound, fetal heart rate monitoring, non-stress tests, and biophysical profiles.

The sixth chapter discusses labor and delivery, including the induction of labor and the manner of delivery. The chapter also covers postpartum care for diabetic women.

Chapter Seven discusses postpartum blood sugar control and medication management while breastfeeding. The chapter also discusses aftercare and contraceptive choices.

Finally, chapter eight discusses long-term diabetes treatment, such as future pregnancy planning and emotional and mental health concerns.

Overall, this book is an excellent resource for controlling fetal distress syndrome. The chapter also goes into how to diagnose and handle these issues.

Diabetes during pregnancy, with an emphasis on improving outcomes for both mother and child. The book offers practical advice and direction to healthcare providers who work with diabetic women, as well as to diabetic women who are planning or are currently pregnant.

1

What Exactly is Diabetes?

Diabetes is classified into numerous forms, including type 1, type 2, gestational diabetes, and other less common varieties. Type 1 diabetes is an autoimmune disease in which the body's immune system assaults and destroys the pancreas. The most prevalent type of diabetes is type 2 diabetes, which arises when the body becomes immune to insulin or does not produce enough insulin to meet the body's needs. Gestational diabetes is a kind of diabetes that develops during pregnancy and normally resolves after the baby is born. Monogenic diabetes and cystic fibrosis-related diabetes are two less prevalent kinds of diabetes.

If untreated, high blood sugar levels can lead to a variety of health issues, including damage to the eyes, kidneys, nerves, and blood vessels. Diabetes can also increase the risk of cardiovascular disease, stroke, and other disorders. High blood sugar levels in pregnant women with diabetes can harm both the mother and the growing fetus. Therefore, to lessen the risk of problems, blood sugar levels must be managed during pregnancy.

Diabetes Types During Pregnancy

Diabetes can manifest itself in three ways during pregnancy:

Gestational Diabetes

This is the most common kind of gestational diabetes, affecting around 6% to 9% of all pregnancies. When the body is unable to manufacture enough insulin to satisfy the increasing demands of pregnancy, gestational diabetes develops. This kind of diabetes normally goes away after delivery, but women who get it are more likely to develop type 2 diabetes later in life.

Type 1 Diabetes

This is an autoimmune illness in which the body's immune system targets and destroys insulin-producing cells in the pancreas. This kind of diabetes is less common. It is most commonly diagnosed before pregnancy. When a woman with type 1 diabetes becomes pregnant, she must carefully manage her blood sugar levels to limit the risk of complications for both herself and the developing fetus.

Type 2 Diabetes

Arises when the body develops insulin resistance or fails to produce enough insulin to meet the body's needs. This kind of diabetes is becoming more common during pregnancy, particularly in overweight or obese women. When a woman with type 2 diabetes becomes pregnant, she must carefully manage her blood sugar levels to limit the risk of complications for both herself and the developing fetus.

The Impact of Diabetes on Pregnancy

Diabetes can have a variety of effects on pregnancy.

• High blood sugar levels in early pregnancy can raise the chance of birth abnormalities, particularly those affecting the heart, brain, and spine.

• High blood sugar levels can cause the infant to grow excessively large: a condition known as macrosomia. A big baby can complicate delivery and increase the risk of injury to both the infant and the mother during labor.

- Diabetes raises the risk of developing pre-eclampsia, a dangerous complication that can harm both the mother and the baby. Pre-eclampsia can result in high blood pressure, protein in the urine, and organ damage, particularly to the kidneys and liver.

- Diabetes increases the risk of preterm delivery, with a higher risk of giving birth prematurely, before 37 weeks.

- If the mother's blood sugar levels are excessively high during pregnancy, the baby's body may create more insulin to compensate. When the infant no longer receives high quantities of glucose from the mother after delivery, his or her blood sugar levels might fall dangerously low, resulting in a condition known as neonatal hypoglycemia.

- Diabetes increases the risk of stillbirth: Diabetes increases the chance of stillbirth, especially if blood sugar levels are inadequately controlled throughout pregnancy.

It is critical for diabetic pregnant women to properly regulate their blood sugar levels during their pregnancy to avoid the risk of complications for both themselves and the growing fetus.

2

Preconception Planning

The process of preparing for pregnancy before fertilization is known as preconception planning. Preconception preparation is crucial for diabetic women who want to have the greatest pregnancy possible. Before becoming pregnant, it is necessary to engage with a healthcare team to optimize blood sugar control, alter medications, and handle any other health risks. Women with diabetes can lower their risk of difficulties and have a healthier pregnancy and infant by taking the required actions to prepare for pregnancy.

The Significance of Preconception Planning

Preconception planning is essential for diabetic women who want to get pregnant since it provides optimal glucose control before conception. Preconception glycemic management has been found to minimize the risk of pregnancy problems and fetal abnormalities are risks. It also reduces the likelihood of maternal problems like hypertension, nephritis, and retinopathy. Furthermore, preconception planning allows healthcare providers to educate women on the importance of glycemic management and change medications and insulin regimens as needed. Women with diabetes can improve their chances of a healthy pregnancy and infant by optimizing their glycemic management before pregnancy.

Counseling Before Conception

Preconception counseling is a type of healthcare that focuses on educating, guiding, and supporting women and their partners before they conceive. The goal of this counseling is to optimize the woman's and her future baby's health before conception. Healthcare providers may discuss preconception counseling with patients. Medical history, lifestyle habits, family planning, medications, and hereditary risks are among the subjects covered. They may also advise on appropriate eating choices, regular exercise, weight management, and stress reduction techniques.

Preconception counseling is important because it can identify and manage any health conditions that may affect pregnancy outcomes, such as diabetes. Preconception counseling assists diabetic women in understanding how their disease may affect pregnancy and how to manage it effectively to reduce potential hazards.

Furthermore, preconception counseling assists women and their partners in making informed reproductive health decisions, such as family planning and contraception. It also allows women to receive assistance and counseling on any emotional or mental health challenges they may be dealing with. Preconception counseling is a critical component of diabetes management in women of reproductive age. It can assist diabetic women to achieve better pregnancy outcomes, minimize the likelihood of problems, and enhance their babies' health.

Pregnancy Blood Sugar Management

Blood sugar control before pregnancy is an important part of preconception planning for diabetic women. Maintaining good blood sugar levels before conception can help lower the chance of birth abnormalities, miscarriage, and other pregnancy issues. High blood sugar levels can harm the growing fetus, especially in the first few weeks of pregnancy when vital organs are developing.

Women with diabetes who wish to become pregnant should work closely with their healthcare professionals to build a specific blood glucose management strategy. Sugar management. This approach may include medication changes, dietary and activity changes, and frequent blood sugar monitoring.

Before becoming pregnant, women should strive for an A1C score of less than 6.5%. This can be accomplished by a mix of dietary and pharmaceutical changes. Women may also be advised to take folic acid supplements before and during pregnancy to help lower the chance of birth abnormalities. Overall, adequate blood sugar control before pregnancy is critical for both the mother's and the growing fetus's health. Preconception planning and counseling can assist diabetic women in preparing for a healthy pregnancy and lowering the chance of problems.

Medication Administration

Medication management is part of preconception planning. Before pregnancy, ensure that your blood sugar levels are under control. If a diabetic woman is using medications to control her blood sugar, she may need to change her treatment regimen before becoming pregnant.

Women who use insulin or oral drugs to control their blood sugar levels may need to change their medication dosages before pregnancy to obtain ideal blood sugar levels. High blood sugar levels during pregnancy can raise the risk of birth abnormalities, premature birth, and other issues.

Furthermore, several drugs routinely used to treat diabetes may be unsafe to take during pregnancy. Some oral diabetic medicines like insulin, for example, may raise the chance of birth abnormalities or other issues. As a result, it is critical for diabetic women to collaborate closely with their healthcare providers to design a medication regimen that is both safe and effective for preconception planning. This may entail changing medications, increasing drug dosages, or making other modifications to ensure that blood sugar levels are well-controlled before becoming pregnant.

3

Pregnancy Blood Sugar Control During Pregnancy

Monitoring Blood Sugar Levels

This is an important element of diabetes management during pregnancy. It contributes to keeping blood sugar levels within a safe range for both the mother and the developing fetus. This chapter will go through the various blood sugar monitoring methods accessible during pregnancy.

SMBG is an abbreviation for Self-Monitoring of Blood Glucose.

- Exactly what is SMBG?

- How to perform SMBG

- When should blood sugar levels be checked?

- Blood sugar levels to aim for during pregnancy

- Keeping track of blood sugar levels

CGM stands for continuous glucose monitoring

- What precisely is CGM?

- How does CGM work?

- Benefits of CGM During Pregnancy

- CGM allows you to control your blood sugar levels.

- CGM restrictions

- Glycated Hemoglobin (HbA1c)

What exactly is HbA1c?

- What role does HbA1c play in blood sugar control?

- When is HbA1c testing performed during pregnancy?

- HbA1c values to aim for during pregnancy

- HbA1c Factors Affecting Blood Sugar Levels During Pregnancy Have Limitations

Changes in hormones during pregnancy

- Insulin sensitivity changes

- Dietary and nutritional requirements

- Physical exercise and activity

- Illness and stress

The Importance of Pregnancy Blood Sugar Monitoring

- Uncontrolled blood sugar levels during pregnancy pose risks.

- Advantages of Keeping Target Blood Sugar Levels During Pregnancy

- The role of healthcare professionals in pregnant blood sugar monitoring

- Tips for Successful Pregnancy Blood Sugar Monitoring

Collaboration with a healthcare team

- Keeping track of your blood sugar levels

- Detecting trends and modifying treatment

- Addressing concerns and difficulties

- Conclusion

The significance of blood sugar monitoring in the management of diabetes during pregnancy

- The various blood sugar monitoring methods available

- Suggestions for Successful Pregnancy blood sugar monitoring

What Exactly is SMBG?

Self-Monitoring of Blood Glucose (SMBG) is a method of self-monitoring blood sugar levels with a glucose meter and test strips. Pricking the fingertip with a lancet to take a little drop of blood, which is then placed on a test strip and injected into a glucose meter, is the procedure for SMBG. After that, the glucose meter measures the amount of glucose in the blood sample and displays the result on the meter's screen.

For patients with diabetes, especially pregnant women, SMBG is a frequent form of blood sugar monitoring. It enables frequent blood sugar checks throughout the day, which can aid with identifying high or low blood sugar levels and adjusting treatment as needed. Diabetes in pregnant women Depending on their unique treatment plan, they may need to conduct SMBG numerous times per day.

SMBG can be performed at home or in a healthcare facility, and it is critical for diabetic pregnant women to follow their healthcare provider's advice on when and how frequently to monitor their blood sugar levels. Keeping a record of blood sugar readings can assist in identifying patterns and making treatment adjustments as needed.

How to Carry out SMBG

Here's a quick rundown on how to do SMBG:

•	Hands should be washed with soap and warm water. They must be fully dried.

•	Prepare the glucose meter and test strip as directed by the manufacturer.

•	Using a lancet, prick the side of your fingertip. Each time, use a different finger to Soreness and calluses should be avoided.

•	Squeeze your finger gently to collect a small drop of blood.

•	Insert the test strip into the glucose meter after placing the blood drop on it.

•	Wait for the blood sugar level to be displayed by the glucose meter. When the test is finished, some meters beep or vibrate.

- Keep track of your blood sugar levels in a logbook or with a smartphone app.

- Dispose of the lancet and test strip as directed by your healthcare provider.

It is critical to follow the directions for the glucose meter and test strips that are being used. Some meters may require a larger blood sample, while others may require a different method of inserting the test strip. Diabetes pregnant women should collaborate closely with their healthcare practitioner to establish how frequently SMBG should be performed and what their target blood sugar levels should be.

When should Blood Sugar Levels Be Checked?

The frequency of blood sugar testing during pregnancy varies according to the type of diabetes, the treatment strategy, and the individual's health. Pregnant women with diabetes should consult with their healthcare professional to decide how frequently their blood sugar levels should be checked.

Here are some general guidelines for when it is appropriate to check blood sugar levels:

- Type 1 diabetes requires women to monitor their blood sugar levels 4 to 8 times per day, including before and after meals, at bedtime, and during the night.

- Women with type 2 diabetes may need to have their blood sugar levels checked 1 to 2 times each day, or as directed by their healthcare physician.

- Women with gestational diabetes may need to monitor their blood sugar levels four to six times each day, including before and after meals.

- Insulin therapy: Women who use insulin may need to monitor their blood sugar levels more frequently than their healthcare physician recommends.

- High-risk pregnancy: Women who have poorly controlled diabetes or other medical disorders may need to check their blood sugar levels more regularly during their pregnancy.

It is critical for diabetic pregnant women to follow their healthcare provider's advice on when to monitor their blood sugar levels

Target Blood Sugar Levels During Pregnancy

Maintaining good blood sugar levels throughout pregnancy is critical for the mother's and baby's health and well-being. Target blood sugar levels for women with preexisting diabetes or gestational diabetes are often lower than for non-pregnant women with diabetes. The American Diabetes Association (ADA) advises the following blood sugar levels for diabetic pregnant women:

- The Blood glucose level at fasting: less than 95 mg/dL

- 1 hour postprandial (after a meal) a blood glucose level of less than 140 mg/dL

- 2-hour postprandial (after meal) a blood glucose level of less than 120 mg/dL

These targets may differ depending on individual circumstances and medical history; therefore, it is critical to collaborate with a healthcare provider to determine suitable blood sugar objectives and develop a treatment plan for a pregnancy diabetes management plan that is unique to you. Maintaining appropriate blood sugar levels through proper diet, frequent physical exercise, and medication control can help reduce difficulties for both the mother and the infant.

Keeping Track of your Blood Sugar Levels

Pregnant women with diabetes and their healthcare providers can make informed decisions regarding medication dosages, diet planning, and exercise routines based on blood sugar readings. Treatment can be adjusted to assist keep blood sugar levels within the target range.

- **Track your progress**: Keeping track of your blood sugar levels over time can help you track your progress and see improvements in your blood sugar control. This can encourage diabetic pregnant women to stick to their treatment plan.

- **Disseminate information**: Pregnant women with diabetes who record their blood sugar levels can discuss their findings with their healthcare provider. This can aid in identifying any areas of concern and adjusting the treatment approach as needed.

Overall, blood sugar monitoring is a useful tool for pregnant women with diabetes in order to control their disease and provide the best potential health results for themselves and their children.

What Exactly Is CGM?

CGM is an abbreviation for Continuous Glucose Monitoring.

It is a sort of glucose monitoring technology that enables continuous real-time measurement of blood sugar levels. CGM is a tiny sensor inserted beneath the skin that continually analyzes the glucose levels in the interstitial fluid (fluid between cells) during the day and night.

The sensor wirelessly delivers data to a receiver or smartphone app, where it may be evaluated to monitor blood sugar changes and make treatment plan adjustments. Some CGM systems additionally include alerts that can notify the wearer when blood sugar levels are abnormally high or low. People with diabetes who need to monitor their blood sugar levels frequently, such as pregnant women or those on insulin therapy, frequently use CGM systems. CGM devices can provide more specific information about blood sugar levels than typical SMBG methods and can assist discover trends in blood sugar levels that intermittent SMBG testing may miss.

Overall, CGM technology has the potential to improve diabetes treatment during pregnancy by providing deeper insight into blood sugar levels. However, working with a healthcare provider to determine if CGM is appropriate and receiving proper training on how to use the system is critical.

How Does CGM Function?

CGM (Continuous Glucose Monitoring) is accomplished by inserting a small sensor beneath the skin, commonly on the abdomen, upper arm, or thigh. The sensor continuously monitors glucose levels in the interstitial fluid, which surrounds the cells in the body.

The CGM sensor is made up of a small, flexible needle injected into the skin and a small transmitter linked to the needle. The glucose measurements are wirelessly transmitted by the transmitter to a receiver or smartphone app The glucose readings are then shown in real-time by the receiver or smartphone app.

CGM systems can offer glucose measurements every few minutes, and some systems can also alert the wearer when glucose levels are too high or too low. Some CGM systems can also predict future glucose trends based on current readings, which is useful for diabetes management.

People with diabetes who need to monitor their glucose levels frequently, such as pregnant women or those on insulin therapy, can use CGM systems. CGM technology can provide more specific information regarding glucose levels than standard self-monitoring of blood glucose (SMBG) methods and can help uncover glucose level trends that intermittent SMBG testing may miss.

CGM systems monitor glucose levels in the interstitial fluid using a tiny electrical current. The current reacts with an enzyme in the sensor that degrades glucose, resulting in an electrical signal that is sent to the receiver. It is crucial to highlight that CGM devices supplement rather than replace standard SMBG approaches. Pregnant women with diabetes should consult with their doctor to decide whether CGM is appropriate for them and to obtain sufficient training on how to use the system.

CGM Advantages during Pregnancy

CGM (continuous glucose monitoring) can provide various advantages for diabetic pregnant women. Here are some of the potential advantages of using CGM during pregnancy:

Improved glucose control: Because CGM can provide real-time feedback on glucose levels, diabetic pregnant women can make prompt changes to their treatment plans. This can result in improved glucose control and a lower risk of pregnancy problems.

Fewer hypoglycemic episodes: CGM systems can notify diabetic pregnant women when their glucose levels are too low, which might help prevent hypoglycemic episodes. Hypoglycemia is especially harmful during pregnancy since it can harm the fetus.

Identifying glucose patterns: CGM technology can detect glucose trends that standard SMBG methods may overlook. This information can assist diabetic pregnant women and their healthcare professionals in adjusting their treatment plans to better regulate their glucose levels.

Reducing stress and anxiety: CGM can give pregnant women with diabetes with peace of mind by allowing them to conveniently monitor their glucose levels without the need for repeated finger tests. This can aid in the reduction of tension and anxiety during pregnancy.

Improved pregnancy outcomes: CGM can help lower the risk of pregnancy problems by delivering more detailed information regarding glucose levels. Pregnancy problems linked with uncontrolled diabetes, such as pre-eclampsia, early birth, and fetal discomfort, can be reduced using CGM.

Overall, CGM can be a useful tool for diabetic pregnant women to manage their condition and ensure the best possible health outcomes for themselves and their babies. However, working with a healthcare provider to determine if CGM is appropriate and receiving proper training on how to use the system is critical.

CGM Allows You to Control Your Blood Sugar Levels

Target blood sugar levels for diabetic pregnant women utilizing CGM (Continuous Glucose Monitoring) may differ depending on individual characteristics such as diabetes type, pre-pregnancy glucose control, and other medical problems.

In general, the blood sugar targets listed below are:

- Blood sugar levels after fasting: 95 mg/dL (5.3 mmol/L) or less

- One hour after a meal, blood sugar levels are as follows: 140 mg/dL (7.8 mmol/L) or less

- Two hours after a meal, blood sugar levels are as follows: 120 mg/dL (6.7 mmol/L) or less

These goals are based on the American Diabetes Association's (ADA) and the International Society for Pediatric and Adolescent Diabetes (ISPAD) recommendations. Pregnant women with diabetes, on the other hand, should consult with their healthcare physician to identify their unique target blood sugar levels.

It is vital to highlight that CGM technology delivers real-time input on glucose levels, which can help diabetic pregnant women adapt their treatment plan to keep glucose levels within the target range. Diabetes pregnant women should collaborate with their healthcare physician to establish a customized treatment strategy that takes into account their specific needs and goals for glucose control.

CGM Restrictions

While CGM (continuous glucose monitoring) technology has many advantages for diabetic pregnant women, there are some drawbacks to consider. Here are some of the potential drawbacks of using CGM:

Cost: CGM systems can be costly, and they may not be covered by insurance for everyone. This may make them less accessible to some diabetic pregnant women

Accuracy: CGM systems are not always 100 percent accurate, and glucose levels may vary. This can result in false alarms or missing hypoglycemia or hyperglycemia events.

Calibration: CGM systems must be calibrated on a regular basis using fingerstick blood glucose testing, which can be time-consuming and inconvenient.

Technical concerns: sensor faults, data transmission issues, or software malfunctions can occur with CGM systems. This can result in missed or incorrect glucose readings.

Skin irritation: Because CGM sensors are implanted beneath the skin, some pregnant women may experience skin irritation or discomfort.

Pregnant women who use CGM must be appropriately educated and taught how to utilize the system, interpret glucose levels, and alter their treatment plans accordingly.

Overall, while CGM technology can be a valuable tool for diabetic pregnant women, it is critical to consider these limitations, and work with a healthcare provider to determine if CGM is appropriate for you to receive proper training on how to use the system.

What Really is HbA1c?

HbA1c, commonly known as A1c, is a blood test that determines the average blood glucose (sugar) levels during the previous two to three months. Rather than a snapshot of a particular moment in time, it provides an overall picture of how effectively a person's blood sugar has been controlled over time.

HbA1c is a blood test that evaluates the quantity of glycated hemoglobin in the blood. Hemoglobin is said to be a protein found in red blood cells that transport oxygen throughout the body. It becomes glycated when exposed to high quantities of glucose in the blood. Because the amount of glycated hemoglobin in the blood is directly proportional to the amount of glucose in the blood, measuring HbA1c can provide an estimate of a person's average blood glucose levels over time. HbA1c is measured as a percentage of total hemoglobin and has a normal range of 4% to 5.6%. The American Diabetes Association (ADA) advises an HbA1c target of less than 7% for most people with diabetes and personalized objectives based on age, duration of diabetes, and other characteristics for some people. HbA1c testing is an important tool for evaluating diabetes care and making necessary changes to treatment programs.

What role does HbA1c play in blood sugar control?

HbA1c measures the quantity of glycated hemoglobin in the blood, which is directly related to the amount of glucose in the blood over the previous 2 to 3 months and hence represents blood sugar control. When blood sugar levels are high, more hemoglobin is glycated, resulting in anemia.

When is HbA1c testing performed during pregnancy?

HbA1c testing during pregnancy may differ depending on the preferences of the healthcare provider and the particular patient's medical history. However, HbA1c testing is generally recommended as part of routine diabetes management during the first trimester of pregnancy.

HbA1c testing may be performed prior to conception for women with preexisting diabetes who are planning to become pregnant or have recently learned that they are pregnant to monitor blood sugar management and make any required adjustments to the treatment plan. During pregnancy, HbA1c levels may be checked on a regular basis, such as every 4-6 weeks, to ensure that blood sugar levels are stable. Patients can collaborate to regulate blood sugar levels and lower the risk of diabetic complications.

Pre-eclampsia, premature birth, macrosomia (big babies), and neonatal hypoglycemia have all been linked to high HbA1c levels during pregnancy. As a result, close monitoring of blood sugar levels, including HbA1c, is critical for diabetes management during pregnancy.

HbA1c values can be influenced by variables such as anemia, hemoglobinopathy, and chronic renal disease, resulting in artificially high or low findings. Alternative blood sugar control measures, such as self-monitoring of blood glucose levels or continuous glucose monitoring, may be used in conjunction with insulin in some cases. HbA1c testing provides a more comprehensive picture of blood sugar control throughout pregnancy.

Hba1c Values to Aim for During Pregnancy

The goal HbA1c levels during pregnancy may differ depending on the particular patient's medical history and the preferences of the healthcare provider. However, the American Diabetes Association recommends a target HbA1c level of less than 6% for diabetic pregnant women. This is less than 7%, which is the suggested target for non-pregnant individuals.

Maintaining HbA1c levels within this target range is critical for blood sugar management and lowering the risk of problems for both the mother and the infant. Pre-eclampsia, premature birth, macrosomia (big baby), and neonatal hypoglycemia have all been linked to high HbA1c levels during pregnancy. It is crucial to highlight that achieving goal HbA1c levels during pregnancy might be difficult, as blood sugar levels may be more difficult to regulate due to hormonal changes. Close monitoring of blood sugar levels, regular prenatal care, and making necessary adjustments to the treatment plan is critical for managing diabetes during pregnancy and decreasing the risk of problems.

HbA1c Limitations

While HbA1c testing is a useful tool for tracking blood sugar control over time, HbA1c has some drawbacks

Alterations: HbA1c values may be altered by variables such as anemia, hemoglobinopathy, and chronic renal disease, resulting in falsely high or low findings in some populations and making it difficult to interpret HbA1c values in certain groups and may necessitate additional blood sugar control methods.

Short-term Sensitivity: HbA1c readings represent blood sugar control over the previous 2 to 3 months, which may not catch short-term changes in blood sugar levels. This means that HbA1c testing may be unable to detect rapid changes in blood sugar management, such as those caused by illness or prescription changes.

Lack of Standardization: HbA1c values may differ slightly between laboratories or testing methodologies. This can make comparing data across healthcare providers or using HbA1c as a reliable indicator of blood sugar control challenging.

Certain conditions limit its utility: HbA1c testing may be performed for all diabetic patients, including those with particular medical conditions or who are pregnant. Alternative blood sugar control measures, such as self-monitoring of blood glucose levels or continuous glucose monitoring, may be used instead in these cases.

Despite these limitations, HbA1c testing remains an important tool in many patients for monitoring blood sugar control and guiding diabetes management. However, healthcare providers should be aware of these limitations and employ additional blood sugar control measures as needed to ensure optimal diabetes management.

Factors Influencing Blood Sugar Levels During Pregnancy Include Hormonal Changes

Hormonal changes during pregnancy can have a major effect on blood sugar levels in diabetic women. Some of the most important hormonal changes that can alter blood sugar levels are:

Human placental lactogen (HPL) HPL is a pregnancy hormone generated by the placenta. HPL can lead to insulin resistance, which implies that cells in the body may not respond as well to insulin. This can result in elevated blood sugar levels.

Progesterone is a hormone that aids in the maintenance of a healthy pregnancy. It can, however, cause the body to become more resistant to insulin, resulting in greater blood sugar levels.

Estrogen is another hormone that can promote insulin resistance during pregnancy. It can also impact how the liver processes glucose, leading to increased blood sugar levels.

Cortisol is a stress hormone that is produced in the body. Cortisol levels may be higher than normal during pregnancy, contributing to higher blood sugar levels.

Glucagon is a hormone that causes the liver to release glucose into the bloodstream, hence raising blood sugar levels. Glucagon levels may be higher than normal during pregnancy, contributing to higher blood sugar levels.

These hormonal changes can make it more difficult for diabetic women to keep their blood sugar levels under control during pregnancy. Blood sugar levels are closely monitored, prenatal care is provided regularly, and treatment plans are adjusted as appropriate.

Insulin Sensitivity

Insulin sensitivity might change during pregnancy, affecting blood sugar levels in diabetic women. Insulin sensitivity may rise during the first trimester of pregnancy, which indicates that the body's cells may respond better to insulin. This might cause blood sugar levels to drop, necessitating changes to the treatment strategy to avoid hypoglycemia (low blood sugar).

However, insulin sensitivity may decrease in the second and third trimesters of pregnancy, meaning that the body's cells may not respond as well to insulin. This can cause blood sugar levels to rise, necessitating changes to the treatment strategy to minimize hyperglycemia (high blood sugar), changes in body weight and metabolism during pregnancy, in addition to hormonal changes, might impact insulin sensitivity. As a woman's body weight increases during pregnancy, insulin sensitivity may decrease, making blood sugar control more difficult.

Close monitoring of blood sugar levels, as well as making necessary adjustments to the treatment plan, are critical for managing diabetes during pregnancy and lowering the risk of complications. Pregnant women with diabetes should collaborate closely with their healthcare provider to design a specific treatment plan that accounts for changes in insulin sensitivity that may occur during pregnancy.

Dietary And Nutritional Requirements

Nutrition and food are critical components of diabetes management during pregnancy. A nutritious diet can help regulate blood sugar levels and lower the risk of difficulties for both the mother and the infant.

Some important nutrition and food considerations for diabetic women during pregnancy include:

Carbohydrate Consumption: Carbohydrates are the body's primary source of energy and can have a substantial impact on blood sugar levels. Women with diabetes who are pregnant may need to carefully regulate their carbohydrate consumption and space out meals and snacks throughout the day to avoid blood sugar increases.

Protein Consumption is essential for fetal growth and development, and it can also aid to manage blood sugar levels. Women with diabetes who are pregnant may require Protein consumption is essential for fetal growth and development, and it can also aid to manage blood sugar levels. Women with diabetes may need to increase their protein intake during pregnancy to ensure that both they and their babies get enough healthy fats, such as those found in nuts, seeds, and

avocados, can be an important element of a healthy diet for pregnant women with diabetes. Saturated and trans fats, on the other hand, should be avoided.

Consumption of fiber: Fiber can help regulate blood sugar levels and promote healthy digestion. Pregnant women with diabetes may need to boost their fiber intake through whole grains, fruits, and vegetables.

Vitamins and Minerals: Pregnant women with diabetes may need to pay extra attention to their consumption of certain vitamins and minerals, such as folic acid, calcium, and iron, to support the baby's health and development.

Balanced and healthy diet rich in whole foods and low in processed and sugary foods is essential for treating diabetes during pregnancy. Women who have diabetes during pregnancy should collaborate with their healthcare physician and a qualified dietitian to create a personalized dietary plan that addresses their specific needs and health goals.

Physical Exercise and Activities

Physical activities and exercise are also essential components of diabetes management during pregnancy. Regular exercise can assist to regulate blood sugar levels, decrease problems, and promote overall health and well-being for both the mother and the infant.

Significant Factors to Consider when it Comes to Physical Activity and Exercise During Pregnancy

Consult with your healthcare provider: Pregnant women with diabetes should consult with their healthcare provider before beginning or changing their exercise regimen to verify that it is safe and appropriate for their unique needs and health status.

Choose low-impact Activities: Low-impact workouts such as walking, swimming, or prenatal yoga can be safe and beneficial options for pregnant women with diabetes. Contact sports and skiing, for example, should be avoided because they pose a significant risk of injury or death.

Monitor Blood Sugar Levels: Pregnant women with diabetes should check their blood sugar levels before and after exercise to ensure they are keeping within their goal range.

Keep Hydrated: Some significant factors to consider when it comes to physical activity and exercise during pregnancy are:

- Drinking plenty of water before, during, and after exercise can aid in the prevention of dehydration and the maintenance of good blood sugar levels.

Be Aware of Signs: Pregnant women with diabetes should be aware of any symptoms of hypoglycemia, such as dizziness, sweating, or confusion, and have a strategy in place to handle them if they occur.

Regular physical activity and exercise can help with diabetes management during pregnancy. Women with diabetes during pregnancy should collaborate with their healthcare physicians to create a personalized fitness plan that addresses their specific needs and health goals.

Illness and Stress

Stress and illness can also have an effect on blood sugar levels, making diabetes management more difficult during pregnancy.

Because stress causes the body to release hormones that raise blood sugar levels, it is critical for women with diabetes to practice stress management techniques such as deep breathing, meditation, or yoga during pregnancy. Women with diabetes who are pregnant should also aim to obtain enough rest and sleep, as this can help to reduce stress and promote good blood sugar levels.

Illnesses, such as the common cold or flu, can cause blood sugar levels to vary. Women with diabetes who are pregnant should take precautions to avoid sickness, such as washing their hands frequently and avoiding smoking. Whenever possible, make contact with sick people. Women with diabetes during pregnancy should work closely with their healthcare provider to check their blood sugar levels and alter their medication or insulin as needed if illness occurs.

In rare circumstances, illness or other causes may necessitate adjustments to medicine or insulin dosages in order to maintain healthy blood sugar levels. Women who have diabetes during pregnancy should work closely with their healthcare provider to monitor their blood sugar levels and, if necessary, change their medication or insulin regimen. To limit the risk of difficulties for both the mother and the baby, it is critical to follow the recommendations and instructions of your healthcare professional when managing diabetes during pregnancy.

The Significance of Blood Sugar Monitoring During Pregnancy: The Dangers of Uncontrolled Blood Sugar Levels During Pregnancy

Blood sugar levels must be monitored during pregnancy for diabetic women to avoid the risk of problems. Uncontrolled blood sugar levels during pregnancy can harm both the mother and the baby. Uncontrolled blood sugar levels during pregnancy can raise the mother's risk of getting preeclampsia, a major pregnancy complication that can include high blood pressure and organ damage such as the liver and kidneys. Uncontrolled blood sugar levels can also raise the risk of infection and impede the healing process after giving birth. Healthy fats such as those found in nuts, and avocados, can be an important element of a healthy diet for pregnant women with diabetes. Saturated and trans fats, on the other hand, should be avoided.

For the baby, uncontrolled blood sugar levels during pregnancy can increase the risk of developing congenital anomalies, such as: heart problems, neural tube defects, and macrosomia, a disease in which the baby grows overly large, are all possibilities. This can complicate delivery and raise the risk of damage to both the mother and the infant. Uncontrolled blood sugar levels during pregnancy can also raise the risk of preterm labor and the infant developing respiratory distress syndrome.

Regular blood sugar monitoring can assist diabetic women during pregnancy in maintaining appropriate blood sugar levels and reducing the risk of problems. This can include self-monitoring blood sugar levels with a glucometer or continuous glucose monitoring (CGM) equipment, as well as regular appointments with a healthcare practitioner to evaluate blood sugar levels and alter treatment programs as necessary.

Overall, blood sugar monitoring Managing diabetes, and decreasing the risk of problems for both the mother and the baby is crucial during pregnancy. Women with diabetes during pregnancy should collaborate closely with their healthcare practitioners to build a personalized monitoring and treatment strategy that takes their specific requirements and health objectives into account.

Advantages of Keeping Target Blood Sugar Levels During Pregnancy

Maintaining target blood sugar levels throughout pregnancy is critical for both the mother's and the baby's well-being. Among the advantages of maintaining good blood sugar levels during pregnancy are:

Preventing problems: Women with diabetes who maintain acceptable blood sugar levels during pregnancy can minimize their chance of developing complications such as preeclampsia, gestational hypertension, and premature labor. Maintaining good health, managing diabetes, and decreasing the risk of problems for both the mother and the baby is crucial during pregnancy. Women with diabetes should work closely with their healthcare provider during pregnancy since blood sugar levels can minimize the risk of infection and slow the healing process after birth.

Maintaining good blood sugar levels during pregnancy can lower the chance of congenital malformations in the infant, such as heart defects or neural tube defects.

Reducing the Risk of Macrosomia: During pregnancy, high blood sugar levels can contribute to macrosomia, a condition in which the baby grows abnormally large. This can make labor more difficult and raise the risk of damage to both the mother and the baby. Keeping blood sugar levels in check can help lower the risk of macrosomia. Maintaining healthy blood sugar levels throughout pregnancy can enhance fetal outcomes, such as lowering the chance of stillbirth and enhancing neonatal outcomes.

Improving maternal outcomes: Women who maintain good blood sugar levels during pregnancy may have fewer difficulties during delivery and a shorter postpartum recovery period.

Overall, maintaining healthy blood sugar levels during pregnancy is critical for both the mother's and the baby's health. Women who have diabetes throughout pregnancy should work closely with their healthcare practitioner to build a specific monitoring and treatment strategy that will assist them in maintaining appropriate blood sugar levels throughout their pregnancy.

The Role of Healthcare Professionals in Pregnancy Blood Sugar Monitoring

Healthcare providers play an important role in diabetic women's blood sugar monitoring throughout pregnancy. They collaborate with pregnant women to create tailored monitoring and treatment regimens to assist them in maintaining appropriate blood sugar levels during their pregnancy. Here are some specific roles that healthcare professionals play in pregnancy blood sugar monitoring:

Creating a Monitoring and Treatment Plan:
Obstetricians, endocrinologists, and trained diabetes educators collaborate with pregnant women to create tailored monitoring and treatment plans based on their unique health needs and diabetes control goals.

Educating pregnant women on blood sugar monitoring: Healthcare providers educate pregnant women on how to check their blood sugar levels, which includes:

- How often to test, what blood sugar levels to strive for, and how to record their results.

- Blood sugar data review: Healthcare experts analyze blood sugar data on a regular basis to ensure that pregnant women maintain healthy blood sugar levels and make any required adjustments to their treatment plans.

Medication Adjustments: Based on blood sugar levels and other factors such as weight growth and physical activity, healthcare experts may need to change medications such as insulin or oral hypoglycemic agents.

Emotional Assistance: Healthcare professionals also provide emotional support to diabetic pregnant women, who may feel greater stress and anxiety during pregnancy due to the additional demands of blood sugar monitoring and management.

Healthcare professionals play an important role in blood sugar monitoring. During pregnancy, diabetes education, monitoring, medication adjustments, and emotional support are provided to help women with diabetes maintain healthy blood sugar levels throughout their pregnancy.

Working With a Healthcare Team; Tips for Successful Blood Sugar Monitoring During Pregnancy

Monitoring blood sugar levels during pregnancy involves a collaborative effort between pregnant women with diabetes and their healthcare team. Here are some pointers to aid with blood sugar monitoring throughout pregnancy:

Form a relationship with your healthcare team: Develop a customized monitoring and treatment strategy with your healthcare team based on your particular health needs and diabetes management goals.

Recognize your blood sugar targets: Make sure you understand your target blood sugar levels and how frequently you should monitor them

levels in order to meet their goals: Consider employing technology, such as a continuous glucose monitor

(CGM), to help you monitor your blood sugar levels more conveniently and accurately.

Maintain a logbook of your blood sugar levels, medications, and meals: Bring it to your healthcare appointments to discuss with your healthcare team.

Make necessary lifestyle changes: To assist maintain healthy blood sugar levels during pregnancy, adjust your diet and physical activity levels as needed.

Keep track of your medical appointments: Attend all of your medical appointments and follow your healthcare team's blood sugar monitoring and treatment recommendations.

Seek emotional assistance: Pregnancy can be a stressful time, and having diabetes can make it even more so a layer of tension. Seek emotional support from friends, family, and support groups as needed to help you cope with stress and stick to your blood sugar monitoring and treatment plan.

Working together with your healthcare team, routinely checking your blood sugar levels, and making necessary lifestyle adjustments can help you successfully manage your diabetes throughout pregnancy and protect the health of both you and your baby.

Maintaining a Record of Blood Sugar Levels

Keeping track of your blood sugar levels is an important aspect of successfully managing diabetes during pregnancy. It allows you and your healthcare team to track your progress and make changes to your diabetes treatment strategy as needed.

Here are some pointers on how to keep track of your blood sugar levels:

- **Select a logbook or app**: To keep track of your blood sugar readings, meals, medications, and physical exercise, use a logbook or diabetes management software.

- **Record your levels at the recommended intervals**: Your healthcare team will advise you on how frequently to monitor your blood sugar levels. Record your blood sugar readings at the appropriate times, such as before and after meals or before going to bed.

- **Make a note of any changes in your routine**: If you make any modifications to your diabetes management plan, such as modifying your medications or changing your food or physical activity, make a note of it in your logbook or app.

- **Bring your appointment logbook or app**: Bring your logbook or app to your medical appointments so you may discuss your progress with your doctor and make any required changes to your diabetes treatment strategy.

- **Examine your logbook or app frequently**: Reviewing your logbook or app on a regular basis can assist you in identifying patterns or trends in your blood sugar levels and adjusting your diabetes management plan accordingly.

- **Maintain your organization**: Keep your logbook or app structured and up to date to assist you and your healthcare team in managing your condition. You may help ensure the best possible outcomes for you and your baby throughout pregnancy by maintaining a record of your blood sugar readings and other diabetes management information.

Detecting Trends and Modifying Treatment

Keeping track of your blood sugar levels during pregnancy can assist you and your healthcare team in identifying patterns and adjusting your treatment plan as needed. Here are some pointers for recognizing patterns and changing medication based on blood sugar monitoring:

Keep an eye out for trends: Examine your blood sugar diary or app on a regular basis for patterns in your blood sugar levels. For example, if you routinely experience high blood sugar levels after a particular meal or at a specific time of day, you may need to modify your diet.

Treatment Plan or Drug Regimen

Consult with your medical team: Discuss any patterns or trends you've noticed in your blood sugar diary or app with your healthcare provider. To better manage your blood sugar levels, your healthcare team can assist you in adjusting your diabetes management plan.

Adjust your Treatment Plan: Your healthcare provider may recommend changes to your treatment plan based on the patterns and trends you've discovered. This could include changing your drug regimen, altering your diet, or boosting your physical activity.

Maintain Regular Communication with your Healthcare Team and offer updates on your blood sugar levels as well as any changes to your treatment plan. This might assist in tailoring your diabetes management plan to your specific needs and goals. You can help improve your blood sugar management and lower the risk of problems during pregnancy by identifying patterns and altering your treatment plan depending on your blood sugar monitoring.

Addressing Concerns and Difficulties

Diabetes management during pregnancy might provide a number of difficulties and concerns.

Here are some pointers for dealing with frequent issues and concerns:

Fear of Hypoglycemia: Hypoglycemia, or low blood sugar, can be a concern for pregnant diabetic women to continue to monitor them. Blood sugar levels and chart their progress in their logbook or app after making changes to their treatment plan. This can assist you and your healthcare team in determining to avoid hypoglycemia, it is critical to frequently monitor your blood sugar levels and eat small, frequent meals throughout the day. Discuss with your healthcare provider how to prevent and manage hypoglycemia, such as changing your medication regimen or keeping a fast-acting source of glucose on hand at all times.

Difficulty keeping to a Meal Plan: Maintaining a nutritious diet plan throughout pregnancy can be difficult, especially if you suffer from nausea or food aversions. Develop a meal plan with a qualified dietitian or certified diabetes educator that meets your specific needs and interests. If you're having trouble keeping to your meal plan, try integrating short, healthy snacks throughout the day or altering your meal timing.

Pregnancy Can Cause Emotional Distress. Managing diabetes can add an extra layer of stress to an already stressful situation. Consider speaking with a mental health professional or joining a support group for pregnant women with diabetes. Regular exercise, meditation, and deep breathing techniques can also aid in stress reduction.

Fear of Problems: Pregnant women with diabetes are more likely to experience complications such as pre-eclampsia, preterm labor, and stillbirth. Maintaining good blood sugar management and attending all of your prenatal checkups will help lower your chance of problems. Discuss any concerns you have with your healthcare provider, and work together to build a plan to manage your diabetes and lower your risk of complications, by addressing common problems and challenges, as well as collaborating closely with your healthcare provider to successfully control your diabetes while pregnant while also promoting a healthy pregnancy and birth result.

Insulin Therapy

Important things to know about insulin therapy during pregnancy

Insulin therapy is a common treatment option for women with diabetes during pregnancy. Insulin is said to be a hormone that helps regulate blood sugar levels in the body. In women with diabetes, insulin therapy can help control blood sugar levels and reduce the risk of complications during pregnancy.

Types of Insulin

There are different types of insulin available such as; short-acting, intermediate-acting, rapid-acting and, long-acting insulin. Your healthcare team will work with you to determine the type and dosage of insulin that is right for you.

Insulin Delivery Methods: Insulin can be delivered using a syringe, insulin pen, or insulin pump. Your healthcare team will work with you to determine the best delivery method for your individual needs.

Dosage Adjustments: Insulin dosage may need to be adjusted throughout pregnancy to maintain target blood sugar levels. It's important to monitor blood sugar levels regularly and work closely with your healthcare team to make any necessary adjustments to your insulin regimen.

Hypoglycemia Risk: Insulin therapy can increase the risk of hypoglycemia, or low blood sugar. It's important to monitor blood sugar levels regularly and to carry a fast-acting source of glucose with you at all times.

Gestational Diabetes: Women with gestational diabetes may be able to manage their blood sugar levels with diet and exercise alone, or may require insulin therapy if diet and exercise are not enough to control blood sugar levels. Insulin therapy is an important treatment option for women with diabetes during pregnancy. By working closely with your healthcare team and monitoring blood sugar levels regularly, you can help ensure the safety and health of both you and your baby during pregnancy.

Meal Planning and Nutrition

Meal planning and proper nutrition are important components of managing diabetes during pregnancy. Eating a healthy and balanced diet can help control blood sugar levels, reduce the risk of complications, and support the growth and development of the baby. Here are some tips for meal planning and nutrition during pregnancy with diabetes:

Choose Nutrient-Dense Foods: Focus on eating nutrient-dense foods that provide essential vitamins, minerals, and fiber, such as fruits, vegetables, whole grains, lean protein, and low-fat dairy products.

Watch Portion Sizes: Eating too much of any type of food, even healthy foods, can cause blood sugar levels to spike. It's important to watch portion sizes and eat meals at regular intervals throughout the day.

Count Carbohydrates: Carbohydrates are an important source of energy for the body, but they can also have a significant impact on blood sugar levels. Your healthcare team may recommend counting carbohydrates to help manage blood sugar levels.

Choose Healthy Fats: While fats should be consumed in moderation, it's important to choose healthy fats such as those found in nuts, seeds, avocados, and fatty fish. These can help improve insulin sensitivity and support overall health.

Avoid Processed Foods: Processed foods can be high in sugar, unhealthy fats, and sodium and can cause blood sugar levels to spike. It's best to choose whole, unprocessed foods when possible.

Stay hydrated: Drinking plenty of water is important for overall health and can help control blood sugar levels. Target at least 8-10 glasses of water in a day.

Work with a registered dietitian: A registered dietitian can help create a personalized meal plan that meets your individual needs and preferences, and can provide guidance and support throughout your pregnancy.

Proper nutrition and meal planning are essential components of managing diabetes during pregnancy. By choosing healthy foods, watching portion sizes, and working with a registered dietitian, you can help control blood sugar levels and support the health of both you and your baby.

Exercise During Pregnancy

Exercise during pregnancy can have many benefits for women with diabetes, including helping to control blood sugar levels, improving circulation, reducing the risk of complications, and supporting overall health and well-being. However, it's important to talk to your healthcare team before starting any exercise program to ensure that it's safe and appropriate for your individual needs.

Here are some tips for exercising safely and effectively during pregnancy with diabetes:

Talk to your Healthcare Team: Before starting any exercise program, talk to your healthcare team to determine what type and intensity of exercise is safe and appropriate for your individual needs.

Choose Low-impact Activities: Low-impact activities such as walking, swimming, cycling, and prenatal yoga are generally safe and effective for pregnant women with diabetes.

Monitor Blood Sugar Levels: Exercise can affect blood sugar levels, so it's important to monitor your levels before, during, and after exercise to ensure they stay within a healthy range.

Stay Hydrated: Drink plenty of water before, during, and after exercise to stay hydrated and support proper bodily function.

Wear Comfortable Clothing: Wear loose, comfortable clothing that allows for proper movement and ventilation.

Listen to Your Body: Pay attention to how you feel during exercise and stop immediately if you experience any discomfort or pain.

Avoid Certain Activities: Some activities, such as contact sports, high-impact aerobics, and activities with a risk of falling, should be avoided during pregnancy.

Exercise can be a safe and effective way to manage diabetes during pregnancy, but it's important to talk to your healthcare team and take precautions to ensure that you and your baby stay safe and healthy. By choosing low-impact activities, monitoring blood sugar levels, staying hydrated, wearing comfortable clothing, and listening to your body, you can enjoy the many benefits of exercise during pregnancy.

4

Probable Complications of Diabetes in Pregnancy

Diabetes in pregnancy can increase the risk of certain complications for both the mother and baby.

These are some potential complications that may arise:

Macrosomia: High blood sugar levels can cause the baby to grow larger than normal, a condition called macrosomia. This can increase the risk of complications during delivery and may require a cesarean section.

Hypoglycemia: Low blood sugar levels can occur in the baby after delivery if the mother's blood sugar levels were high during pregnancy, this can cause the baby to have difficulty breathing, seizures, or other health problems.

Pre-eclampsia: Women with diabetes during pregnancy are at increased risk for developing pre-eclampsia, a condition characterized by swelling, protein in the urine, and high blood pressure

Polyhydramnios: Polyhydramnios is a disorder characterized by an abnormally large volume of amniotic fluid around the fetus in the uterus. Normally, the amniotic fluid acts as a protective cushion for the developing fetus, allowing movement and growth while also maintaining a sterile environment. However, if there is an abnormally large amount of amniotic fluid present, it may indicate an underlying problem.

Polyhydramnios can be caused by a variety of factors, including gestational diabetes, hypertension, fetal abnormalities, multiple gestations (twins, triplets, etc.), and maternal medical issues such as maternal heart disease or thyroid disorders. In certain circumstances, the root cause is unknown.

During standard prenatal care, ultrasound imaging can detect polyhydramnios by measuring the amount of amniotic fluid present in the uterus. Mild cases may not result in any symptoms, while more severe cases may result in discomfort, trouble breathing, and swelling in the mother's extremities. Polyhydramnios can raise the risk of pregnancy and delivery difficulties such as preterm labor, premature rupture of the membranes, and placental abruption. It can also raise the likelihood of maternal problems such as postpartum hemorrhage and infection.

Polyhydramnios treatment is determined by the severity and underlying etiology of the disorder. Mild cases may not require treatment; however, severe cases may necessitate amniocentesis (the removal of extra amniotic fluid), induction of labor, or cesarean delivery.

Overall, pregnant women should keep their prenatal checkups and address any concerns or symptoms with their healthcare provider. This can aid in ensuring early detection and care of diseases such as polyhydramnios resulting in improved outcomes for both the mother and the infant.

Gestational Hypertension: Gestational hypertension is characterized by elevated blood pressure during pregnancy. It usually appears after the 20th week of pregnancy and affects 5-10% of pregnancies worldwide. Although the specific origin of gestational hypertension is unknown, it is thought to be related to a problem with the blood arteries that supply the placenta.

Women with gestational hypertension are more likely to develop preeclampsia, a dangerous complication that can cause organ damage and even death if not treated. High blood pressure, proteinuria (extra protein in the urine), and other signs of organ damage, such as headaches, vision abnormalities, and stomach pain, are all symptoms of preeclampsia. Gestational hypertension may also raise the risk of premature birth, low birth weight, and stillbirth. As a result, detecting and managing gestational hypertension early is crucial to ensuring the best possible outcome for both the mother and the baby.

When a woman has high blood pressure (blood pressure equal to or more than 140/90 mm Hg) after the 20th week of pregnancy and no proteinuria or other indications of preeclampsia, she is diagnosed with gestational hypertension. However, some women may experience preeclampsia early in pregnancy or develop proteinuria later in pregnancy, indicating the onset of preeclampsia.

Gestational hypertension is normally managed by closely monitoring blood pressure and fetal well-being, as well as managing any underlying disorders that may contribute to high blood pressure, such as pre-existing hypertension or diabetes.

Depending on the situation, drugs to decrease blood pressure and avoid complications may be administered.

Gestational hypertension is a common illness that, if left untreated, can have catastrophic effects for both the mother and the baby. Early detection and control are critical to achieving the best possible outcome for all parties.

Preterm Labor: Preterm labor can occur naturally or be medically induced. The etiology of preterm labor is unknown in some cases, however, risk factors such as maternal age, smoking, previous preterm birth, uterine anomalies, cervical incompetence, infection, and multiple gestations can all raise the incidence of premature labor.

Preterm labor symptoms may include more than six contractions per hour, lower stomach or back pain, pelvic pain and Pressure, vaginal discharge or bleeding, and a rise in vaginal discharge are all possible symptoms. If a woman has any of these symptoms, she should seek medical assistance right away.

Preterm labor is typically diagnosed by examining the woman's symptoms and completing a physical examination, which includes a pelvic examination to examine the cervix. In some circumstances, tests such as a fetal fibronectin test or a transvaginal ultrasound to measure cervical length may be performed to detect whether preterm labor is impending.

If preterm labor is discovered, the goal of treatment is to postpone birth long enough to allow for adequate fetal outcomes interventions. Treatments may include bed rest, contraction suppressants, and corticosteroids to assist the fetal lung's maturity. Delivery may be delayed in some circumstances if the hazards of extending the pregnancy outweigh the advantages, termination is required. Preventing preterm labor entails identifying and resolving risk factors before pregnancy, receiving frequent prenatal care to check for early signs of preterm labor, and managing conditions such as gestational diabetes and hypertension appropriately. Progesterone supplements during pregnancy may also benefit women who have a history of premature labor or other risk factors for preterm birth.

Birth Defects: Birth defects are physical or functional abnormalities that occur at birth and can be caused by genetic or environmental factors. They can range from mild abnormalities that have no impact on a person's health or quality of life to severe deformities that can be fatal or cause long-term disability. Birth defects can affect many different sections of the body, including the heart, lungs, brain, spine, and limbs. Cleft lip and palate, heart problems, neural tube defects, and Down syndrome are all examples of birth defects.

The causes of birth defects are frequently unknown, but they can be impacted by a number of variables, including genetics, exposure to particular chemicals or illnesses during pregnancy, and environmental factors. Smoking and drug use are examples of lifestyle factors. Some birth abnormalities are inherited from one or both parents, while others develop on their own as a result of a random genetic mutation or environmental exposure.

Early detection and intervention can help treat and prevent many birth abnormalities. Prenatal screening tests and ultrasound can detect potential birth problems, and medical procedures like as surgery or medication may be advised to address specific difficulties. However, birth abnormalities may not be diagnosed until after birth in rare situations, and continued medical care and support may be required throughout a person's life.

Type 2 Diabetes: Women with diabetes in pregnancy are at increased risk of developing type 2 diabetes later in life. It's important to work closely with your healthcare team to monitor and manage your blood sugar levels during pregnancy to help reduce the risk of these and other complications. By controlling blood sugar levels, following a healthy diet and exercise program, and attending all recommended prenatal appointments, you can help ensure the health and well-being of both you and your baby.

Diabetes type 2 is a chronic metabolic condition that affects how the body processes glucose (sugar) in the blood. It is characterized by insulin resistance, which implies that the body is unable to adequately use insulin to regulate blood sugar levels. As a result, blood sugar levels rise, causing a range of health issues.

Type 2 diabetes is the most common type, accounting for almost 90% of all cases. It is primarily diagnosed in adults, but due to increased obesity rates, it is becoming more common in children and adolescents. Being overweight or obese, having a family history of diabetes, and leading a sedentary lifestyle are all risk factors for acquiring type 2 diabetes.

Increased blood sugar levels are one of the symptoms of type 2 diabetes. Thirst, frequent urination, hazy eyesight, weariness, poor wound healing, and tingling or numbness in the hands and feet are all symptoms. However, many people with type 2 diabetes have no symptoms at all, which is why regular blood sugar checks are vital if you are at risk.

Type 2 diabetes treatment often consists of lifestyle changes such as diet and exercise, as well as medications to help regulate blood sugar levels. Insulin therapy may be required in some circumstances.

Type 2 diabetes, if left untreated, can lead to a variety of significant problems, including heart disease, stroke, kidney damage, nerve damage, and blindness. Many patients with type 2 diabetes, however, can live normal lives with good blood sugar monitoring and control. Thirst, frequent urination, hazy eyesight, weariness, poor wound healing, and tingling or numbness in the hands and feet are all symptoms. However, many people with type 2 diabetes have no symptoms at all, which is why regular blood sugar checks are vital if you are at risk of living a long and healthy life.

5

Fetal Monitoring

An Overview of fetal monitoring throughout pregnancy

The significance of prenatal monitoring in diabetes-complicated pregnancies

An overview of fetal monitoring techniques:

- Monitoring with ultrasound

- How does ultrasonography work?

- Ultrasound types used for prenatal monitoring

- When is ultrasonography commonly used during pregnancy?

- How can ultrasound detect diabetes issues during pregnancy?

- Monitoring of the fetal heart rate

- What is fetal heart rate monitoring?

- Fetal heart rate monitoring technique

- When fetal heart rate monitoring is typically used during pregnancy

- What a fetal heart rate monitoring might reveal diabetic problems during pregnancy

Non-stress test (NST)

- What is a non-stress test

- How non-stress test is performed

- What non-stress test results indicate

- How non-stress tests can detect complications related to diabetes in pregnancy?

Biophysical profile (BPP)

- What exactly is a biophysical profile?

- How is a biophysical profile done?

- What do the biophysical profile data imply?

- How can a biophysical profile detect diabetic issues during pregnancy?

CST stands for a contraction stress test.

What exactly is a contraction stress test?

- How the contraction stress test is carried out

- What do the contraction stress test findings mean?

- How a contraction stress test might reveal diabetic problems in pregnancy

Fetal monitoring throughout pregnancy

- The significance of regular fetal monitoring in diabetes-complicated pregnancies

- Collaboration between healthcare practitioners and patients is essential for accurate fetal monitoring.

- Based on fetal monitoring results, potential outcomes, and actions are proposed.

Ultrasounds Of the Fetus

Fetal ultrasonography is a medical imaging technology that creates images of the developing fetus in the womb by using high-frequency sound waves. It is a secure and non-invasive method of monitoring fetal growth, development, and well-being during pregnancy. Fetal ultrasounds can be used to check many aspects of fetal health and development at various stages of pregnancy.

Here are some important facts concerning fetal ultrasounds:

Classification of Fetal ultrasounds

Transabdominal Ultrasound

Creates images of the fetus using a transducer positioned on the abdomen. In early pregnancy, a transducer put into the vagina is used to create images of the fetus.

When Performing Fetal Ultrasounds

First-trimester ultrasounds are performed between 11 and 14 weeks of pregnancy to determine the baby's growth, age, and health.

At 18-20 weeks of pregnancy, a second-trimester ultrasound is conducted to check fetal anatomy, growth, and development.

Third-trimester ultrasound: used in late pregnancy to check fetal growth, position, and development.

Transvaginal Ultrasound

Uses a transducer inserted into the vagina to create images of the fetus in early pregnancy When fetal ultrasounds are performed: First trimester ultrasound: is performed at 11-14 weeks of pregnancy to assess fetal size, age, and health Second trimester ultrasound: performed at 18-20 weeks of pregnancy to assess fetal anatomy, growth, and development Third trimester ultrasound: performed in late pregnancy to assess fetal growth, position, and well-being.

Uses of Fetal Ultrasounds

- Confirming pregnancy and gestational age

- Checking for multiple pregnancies Assessing fetal growth and development

- Detecting fetal abnormalities

- Assessing the placenta and amniotic fluid Guiding procedures such as amniocentesis or fetal blood sampling Safety of fetal ultrasounds

Fetal ultrasound is considered safe and has no known harmful effects on the fetus or the mother when used appropriately. However, unnecessary or prolonged exposure to ultrasound should be avoided.

Benefits of Fetal Ultrasounds

- Fetal ultrasounds can provide valuable information about fetal health and development, and help detect potential complications or abnormalities.
- Early detection and treatment of fetal problems can improve outcomes for both the mother and baby.

Limitations of Fetal Ultrasounds

- Fetal ultrasounds have limitations in detecting certain fetal abnormalities, such as those affecting the brain or spine.

- False positive or false negative results are possible, and further testing or monitoring may be needed to confirm or rule out potential problems.

- Fetal ultrasounds may not detect all possible complications related to diabetes in pregnancy, and additional fetal monitoring may be needed. Importance of fetal monitoring in pregnancies complicated by diabetes

Fetal monitoring is crucial in pregnancies complicated by diabetes as high blood sugar levels can increase the risk of various fetal complications.

Macrosomia

This is a condition where the baby grows too large due to excessive glucose crossing the placenta, leading to an increased risk of birth injuries and difficulties during delivery.

Preterm Delivery

Uncontrolled blood sugar levels may lead to premature delivery, which can increase the risk of respiratory distress syndrome, intraventricular hemorrhage, and other complications.

Stillbirth

Diabetes during pregnancy increases the risk of stillbirth, which is when the baby dies in the womb after 20 weeks of pregnancy.

Birth Defects

Poorly controlled diabetes during pregnancy can increase the risk of birth defects such as heart, neural tube, and kidney defects.

Fetal monitoring helps detect any potential complications early, allowing healthcare providers to intervene and prevent any adverse outcomes.

Overview of Various Fetal Monitoring Techniques

There are several techniques available for fetal monitoring during pregnancy, including

Ultrasound

This is a non-invasive procedure that uses high-frequency sound waves to create images of the fetus, allowing healthcare providers to monitor fetal growth and development.

Non-Stress Test (NST)

This test is performed by placing a monitor on the mother's abdomen to measure fetal heart rate and uterine contractions. It is typically done in the third trimester to evaluate fetal well-being.

Biophysical Profile (BPP)

This test combines ultrasound and NST to evaluate fetal breathing movements, muscle tone, fetal movements, amniotic fluid levels, and fetal heart rate monitoring fetal heart rate patterns in response to uterine contractions induced either naturally or through medication. These monitoring techniques help healthcare providers assess fetal health and detect any potential complications early, allowing for timely interventions to optimize outcomes for both the mother and baby.

Ultrasound Monitoring

Ultrasound monitoring is a non-invasive technique that uses high-frequency sound waves to create images of the fetus, placenta, and amniotic fluid during pregnancy. It is a valuable tool for fetal monitoring as it can provide important information about fetal growth and development, detect structural abnormalities, and evaluate the amount of amniotic fluid.

During ultrasound monitoring, a gel is applied to the mother's abdomen, and a transducer is moved over the skin to send sound waves through the uterus. The sound waves bounce back off the fetus, and the transducer converts them into an image that can be viewed on a monitor.

Types of Ultrasound Scans

Dating Ultrasound: This is typically performed in the first trimester to determine the gestational age of the fetus and estimate the due date.

Anatomy Ultrasound: This is performed in the second trimester to evaluate the fetal anatomy and detect any structural abnormalities.

Growth Ultrasound: This is performed throughout the pregnancy to monitor fetal growth and ensure that the fetus is growing appropriately.

Doppler Ultrasound: This is a specialized type of ultrasound that uses sound waves to evaluate blood flow in the umbilical cord and fetal arteries. Ultrasound monitoring is safe and does not involve radiation, making it a preferred method for fetal monitoring during pregnancy.

How Ultrasound Works

Ultrasound works by using high-frequency sound waves that bounce off the internal structures of the body to create images. During an ultrasound exam, a small handheld device called a transducer is used to emit sound waves into the body.

These sound waves travel through the tissues of the body and bounce back to the transducer, which then creates images of the internal structures on a computer screen. The sound waves used in ultrasound are too high in frequency for humans to hear, and they are safe for both the mother and the fetus.

The ultrasound transducer is usually placed on the mother's abdomen, and a special gel is used to help the sound waves travel through the skin and into the body. As the sound waves travel through the body, they bounce off of different tissues and organs, and the echoes are detected by the transducer. The transducer then sends the information to a computer, which creates an image of the structures inside the body. Ultrasound can be used for a variety of purposes during pregnancy, including determining the gestational age of the fetus, evaluating fetal growth and development, and detecting any structural abnormalities.

It is a safe and non-invasive method of fetal monitoring that provides valuable information for healthcare professionals.

Types of Ultrasounds Used for Fetal Monitoring

There are several types of ultrasounds that may be used for fetal monitoring during pregnancy, including:

Transabdominal Ultrasound: This involves placing the ultrasound transducer on the mother's abdomen to obtain images of the fetus.

Transvaginal Ultrasound: Which involves inserting a small ultrasound transducer into the mother's vagina and issues with blood supply to the fetus.

3D and 4D Ultrasound: offer three-dimensional images of the fetus and can aid in the detection of structural defects or other concerns.

Fetal Echocardiography: This is a form of ultrasound that focuses on the fetus's heart. It can be utilized to discover any abnormalities in the fetal heart's structure or function.

The type of ultrasound utilized for fetal monitoring will be determined by the pregnancy's individual needs and the advice of the healthcare professional.

When Is Ultrasonography Commonly Used During Pregnancy?

During pregnancy, ultrasound is commonly used to examine fetal growth and development, confirm the due date, check the placenta and amniotic fluid levels, and screen for any potential abnormalities. The American College of Obstetricians and Gynecologists (ACOG) suggests at least one complete ultrasound examination around 18 and 22 weeks of pregnancy.

Additional ultrasounds, on the other hand, may be suggested for women with high-risk pregnancies or certain medical issues.

How Ultrasounds Might Detect Diabetic Problems During Pregnancy

Diabetes problems in pregnancy can be detected via ultrasound.

As an example: Diabetes in pregnancy can allow the baby to grow larger than normal, but it can also cause poor fetal growth, which is known as fetal growth restriction. Ultrasound can detect any problems associated with poor fetal growth and evaluate the baby's growth rate and size.

Polyhydramnios: Diabetes patients are at risk of having too much amniotic fluid in their wombs. Polyhydramnios is the medical term for this condition. Ultrasound can detect any abnormalities in amniotic fluid levels.

Diabetes during pregnancy raises the chance of fetal malformations such as neural tube defects and heart disorders. These defects and other possible issues can be detected via ultrasound, allowing for proper monitoring and treatment.

Diabetes can influence the placenta, resulting in placental anomalies including placenta previa, placental insufficiency, and placental abruption. These anomalies can be detected with ultrasound and used to guide appropriate management and therapy.

Overall, ultrasonography is a useful tool for monitoring fetal well-being in diabetes-complicated pregnancies, and it can aid in the identification and management of potential issues.

How To Feel Heart Rate Monitoring During Fetal Life

Monitoring fetal heart rate entails measuring the heart rate of the fetus. A handheld Doppler ultrasonography device or a fetal heart rate monitor can be used for this.

A handheld Doppler ultrasonography instrument detects the fetal heartbeat using high-frequency sound waves. When the gadget is put on the mother's abdomen, sound waves bounce off the fetal heart and return to the device, producing an audible sound. The fetal heart rate can be determined by counting the number of beats per minute.

A fetal heart rate monitor is a more advanced technology that detects the fetal heartbeat using electrodes put on the mother's belly. The electrodes are linked to a machine, which displays the fetal heart rate on a graph or a computer screen. This approach yields a more precise measurement of Fetal heart rate monitoring is typically done during routine prenatal visits and during labor and delivery to detect any potential problems with the fetus, such as fetal distress or abnormalities in the heart rate, which may require further testing or intervention.

Fetal Heart Rate Monitoring Methodology

Fetal heart rate monitoring is classified into two types:

- **External Fetal Heart Rate Monitoring**: This sort of monitoring is performed on the mother's abdomen using an ultrasonography transducer and tocodynamometer. The ultrasound transducer measures fetal heart rate, whereas the tocodynamometer measures contraction frequency and length.

- **Internal Fetal Heart Rate Monitoring**: This sort of monitoring is performed by inserting an electrode via the cervix into the fetal scalp. This approach delivers more accurate readings and allows for continuous monitoring, but it is associated with a higher risk of infection and can only be used during labor.

When Is Fetal Heart Rate Monitoring Commonly Utilized During Pregnancy?

During the third trimester, fetal heart rate monitoring is commonly employed. Beginning around 28 weeks, the third trimester of pregnancy begins. For women with diabetes or other high-risk characteristics, it may be suggested earlier in the pregnancy. During labor, fetal heart rate monitoring is also used to monitor the baby's well-being and to ensure that the infant is tolerating contractions.

What Fetal Heart Rate Monitoring Might Reveal Diabetic Problems During Pregnancy?

By measuring the baby's heart rate and rhythm, fetal heart rate monitoring can aid in the detection of diabetic issues during pregnancy. High blood sugar levels in the mother might induce an erratic heart rhythm in the baby, which can be a symptom of discomfort. If the baby's heart rate is abnormal or he or she exhibits indications of discomfort, more testing may be required to establish the cause and to ascertain whether intervention is required to ensure the baby's well-being. Fetal heart rate monitoring can also detect whether the baby is not growing normally, which can be a consequence of diabetes in pregnancy.

What Exactly is a Non-Stress Test (NST)?

A Non-Stress test (NST) is a non-invasive prenatal monitoring technique that analyzes the fetal heart rate in response to fetal movement. Because there is no stress exerted on the fetus during the test, it is referred to as a "non-stress" test. The test is often performed in a doctor's office or hospital setting and lasts 20 to 30 minutes. Two sensors are inserted in the mother's abdomen during an NST to monitor the fetal heart rate and uterine contractions.

The fetal heart rate is recorded in reaction to fetal movement, which can be either spontaneous or stimulated. To induce fetal movement, the mother may be asked to press a button anytime she feels the baby move, or the doctor may use a device to vibrate the mother's abdomen.

Classification of The NST Results

- **A Reactive Result Indicates** that the fetal heart rate increased in response to fetal movement, indicating that the baby is receiving adequate oxygen and is not in distress.

- **A Non-Reactive Result Indicates** that the fetal heart rate did not raise sufficiently in response to fetal movement, which may suggest that the baby is not getting enough oxygen and that additional testing is required.

How the Non-Stress Test is Carried Out

A healthcare physician will connect two sensors to the pregnant woman's belly during a non-stress test (NST): one to monitor the fetal heart rate and the other to assess contractions. The sensors are linked to a machine that monitors the fetal heart rate as well as any contractions. When the lady feels the baby move, she is instructed to click a button on the equipment. The test normally lasts between 20 and 30 minutes, the healthcare provider will search for accelerations in the fetal heart rate during the examination. Accelerations are brief rises in the fetal heart rate that indicate that the baby is obtaining enough oxygen. If the fetal heart rate does not increase during the test, this could be a symptom of a problem or signs of fetal distress, and more monitoring or intervention may be required.

How A Non-Stress Test Can Detect Diabetes Problems in Pregnancy

A Non-Stress test (NST) is a sort of fetal heart rate monitoring used to assess the fetus's health. The fetal heart rate is monitored during an NST both while the fetus is at rest and when it is active. This is accomplished by implanting a device on the mother's belly that monitors the fetal heart rate and contractions. The test is dubbed a non-stress test since no stress is applied to the fetus during the procedure.

The NST is used to detect diabetic problems in pregnancy, such as fetal distress, which can occur as a result of inadequate diabetes management, controlling blood sugar levels, or other factors. If the fetal heart rate is abnormal or there are signs of distress during the examination, more testing may be required to determine the fetus's health. Early diagnosis of fetal distress can assist healthcare providers in taking the necessary precautions to protect both the mother and the fetus.

A biophysical profile (BPP) is a type of profile that measures the physical properties of a person.

A Biophysical Profile (BPP)

This is a prenatal diagnostic that assesses the fetus's health. The ultrasound and fetal heart rate monitoring used in the test is used to examine the baby's movements, respiration, muscle tone, and amniotic fluid levels. The BPP score ranges from 0 to 10, with 10 being the highest attainable value. The score is calculated thus:

Fetal Breathing Movements: The ultrasound detects the presence or absence of fetal breathing movements.

Fetal Movement: The ultrasound measures how much the fetus moves.

Fetal Tone: The ultrasound evaluates the fetus's muscular tone.

The ultrasound measures the volume of amniotic fluid surrounding the fetus.

Non-stress test for fetal heart rate reactivity: The non-stress test is used to assess the fetal heart rate in reaction to fetal movements. Based on the score, the healthcare provider can assess the fetus's health and determine whether additional monitoring or intervention is required. The BPP is frequently used to monitor fetal well-being in diabetes-complicated pregnancies.

How Is a Biophysical Profile Performed?

A biophysical profile (BPP) is a type of profile A prenatal test that combines an ultrasound examination with a non-stress test (NST) to measure the fetus's well-being. It usually takes between 20 and 40 minutes to complete.

The technician will use a transducer to monitor the fetus's heart rate, respiration, movement, muscle tone, and the amount of amniotic fluid in the uterus during the ultrasound phase of the exam. The technician will also use Doppler ultrasound to assess blood flow in the umbilical cord and fetal brain.

A healthcare provider will place two monitors on the mother's belly during the NST portion of the test to record the fetal heart rate and uterine contractions. The healthcare provider will then assess if the fetal heart rate pattern changes in response to fetal movement and if the fetus is obtaining adequate oxygen and nutrition. Each of the five components tested receives a score based on the findings of the ultrasound and NST portions of the test. The overall score runs from 0 to 10, with a score of 8 to 10 being deemed reassuring and a score of 6 or lower suggesting a potential concern that may necessitate additional testing or intervention.

How Can a Biophysical Profile Detect Diabetic Issues During Pregnancy?

A biophysical profile can aid in the detection of diabetic issues in pregnancy by screening the fetus for evidence of discomfort or compromise in many aspects of its well-being. The fetal breathing motions, fetal body movements, fetal tone, amniotic fluid volume, and fetal heart rate reactivity are all measured.

Diabetes increases the likelihood of various issues, such as fetal abnormalities in pregnancies, growth restriction, fetal discomfort, and stillbirth are all on the rise. A biophysical profile can aid in the early detection of these problems, allowing for appropriate therapies to enhance fetal outcomes. If the biophysical profile reveals indicators of fetal distress, such as decreased fetal movement or a non-reactive fetal heart rate, rapid delivery may be required to protect the fetus from further harm.

Contraction Stress Test (CST)

What Exactly Is the Contraction Stress Test?

A contraction stress test (CST) is a prenatal test that evaluates how the heart rate of a fetus reacts to the stress of contractions. An oxytocin challenge test (OCT) is another name for it. When there is worry about the baby's well-being or when a pregnancy is considered high-risk, the test is frequently conducted.

When performing a CST, the woman's contractions are monitored, and her baby's heart rate is recorded. The purpose of the test is to determine how the baby's heart rate reacts to contractions, which momentarily reduces the amount of oxygen the infant receives. To trigger uterine contractions, a synthetic form of the hormone oxytocin is administered. The purpose is to determine whether the baby's heart rate is steady or if there are any concerning changes that may necessitate more testing or delivery.

How The Contraction Stress Test Is Carried Out

The fetal heart rate is monitored as the uterus is stimulated to contract during a contraction stress test (CST).

There are two methods for stimulating the uterus:

- The healthcare provider stimulates the nipple and may direct the mother to touch her nipples, which produces the hormone oxytocin and induces contractions.

- If nipple stimulation does not result in contractions, the healthcare professional may inject oxytocin, a synthetic type of hormone that causes contractions.

The fetal heart rate is monitored with an electronic fetal monitor during the test. Contractions in the mother are also measured and documented. The test is normally carried out for 10-20 minutes, or until three contractions of sufficient strength and frequency are observed during a 10-minute interval. The test's purpose is to see how the fetus reacts to the stress of the contractions.

If the fetal heart rate remains normal during the test, this is deemed a "negative" result, that the fetus is tolerating the stress of contractions well. If the fetal heart rate is abnormal, it is seen as a "positive" result, meaning that the fetus is not receiving enough oxygen and may need to be delivered. An "equivocal" or "unsatisfactory" result indicates that the test was unable to provide a clear response and that additional testing may be required.

What Does the Contraction Stress Test Show?

The contraction stress test (CST) is used to determine how well the baby will handle the stress of labor and delivery. The fetal heart rate is monitored as the uterus is stimulated to contract during the test. The purpose of the test is to determine whether the baby's heart rate responds adequately to the stress of the situation. contractions.

A negative CST implies that the baby's heart rate remains stable during contractions, which is a strong indication that the infant will cope well with labor and delivery. A positive CST shows that the baby's heart rate does not respond adequately to contractions, which could mean that the baby is not getting enough oxygen throughout labor and delivery. In this instance, more monitoring and intervention may be required to ensure the baby's safety.

How A Contraction Stress Test Might Reveal Diabetic Problems in Pregnancy

The contraction stress test (CST) can detect probable diabetic problems in pregnancy, such as placental insufficiency or fetal distress. The fetus is monitored during a CST for its response to contractions generated by nipple stimulation, or medicine may be used. The idea is to see how the fetus reacts to stress, which can help determine if the fetus receives enough oxygen throughout childbirth.

If the fetus's heart rate decelerates or other irregularities occur during contractions, it may suggest that the fetus is not receiving enough oxygen, which could be due to placental issues. In such instances, the healthcare provider may advise that the infant be delivered.

Review of Fetal Cardiac Monitoring During Pregnancy

The significance of regular fetal monitoring in diabetes-complicated pregnancies

Regular fetal monitoring is essential in diabetes-complicated pregnancies to guarantee the fetus's well-being. Fetal monitoring can detect potential issues caused by diabetes and permits Healthcare experts must act and manage them as soon as possible.

Ultrasound monitoring, fetal heart rate monitoring, a non-stress test (NST), a biophysical profile (BPP), and a contraction stress test (CST) are all possible fetal monitoring techniques. Each approach has advantages and disadvantages and is utilized based on the needs of the pregnancy. Healthcare experts collaborate with the patient to establish which sort of monitoring is best for their specific scenario. Fetal monitoring on a regular basis helps to reduce the risk of fetal problems and ensures that the pregnancy proceeds as smoothly as possible.

Collaboration Between Healthcare Practitioners and Patients

Collaboration between healthcare practitioners and patients is required for effective fetal monitoring. Patients should be educated about the necessity of regular fetal monitoring by healthcare practitioners. Make certain that they have access to the required resources, such as ultrasound equipment and skilled personnel.

Patients, on the other hand, should check their own blood sugar levels and report any changes or concerns to their healthcare professionals. They should also attend all planned fetal monitoring appointments and follow any directions given to them by their healthcare provider. Effective communication between healthcare providers and patients is also essential for fetal monitoring to be successful. Patients should feel free to ask questions and express concerns, and healthcare providers should be attentive and responsive to these issues.

A coordinated approach to fetal monitoring can aid in the early detection of any issues and assure the best possible results for both mother and baby. Based on potential results and interventions based on prenatal monitoring findings

Fetal surveillance throughout pregnancy is critical for recognizing diabetic problems and protecting the health of both the mother and the baby. Various outcomes and treatments may be implemented depending on the results of the fetal monitoring:

Normal fetal monitoring results suggest that the baby is healthy and that there are no immediate concerns. Routine monitoring is maintained in this situation, and no more interventions are required.

Non-reassuring fetal monitoring data indicate that there may be possible issues with the baby's well-being. Depending on the severity of the problem, healthcare providers may advise additional testing, such as a biophysical profile, to obtain additional information. In some circumstances, immediate delivery is required to ensure the baby's safety. Abnormal fetal monitoring results may signal the necessity for rapid delivery to protect the baby's well-being. A C-section may be required in some situations to guarantee the safety of both the mother and the infant.

Ongoing monitoring may be indicated if there are concerns about the baby's well-being but immediate delivery is not required. More frequent ultrasounds or non-stress testing may be required to closely check the baby's health. In any situation, close collaboration between healthcare practitioners and patients is critical to ensuring the greatest outcomes for both mother and infant. It is critical for patients to share any concerns or questions with their healthcare team and to adhere to all suggested monitoring and treatment protocols.

6

Labor And Delivery

Labor Induction

Women with diabetes go through labor and delivery in the same way as women without diabetes. Diabetes, on the other hand, might raise the risk of problems during labor and delivery, necessitating careful monitoring and control.

Induction of labor, which is the act of artificially initiating labor, is one intervention that may be explored for diabetic women. Induction may be advised for a variety of reasons:

•   If the woman has gestational diabetes and finds it difficult to control her blood sugar levels despite diet and exercise, or if her due date has passed.

•   If the woman has diabetes and her baby is expected to be large, or if there are worries about the infant's health and well-being.

•   If the woman has diabetes-related difficulties, such as high blood pressure or kidney problems, it is preferable to have the baby sooner rather than later.

Induction of labor is usually performed in a hospital under the supervision of a healthcare expert. Several steps may be involved in the process, including:

Cervical Ripening is the softening and thinning of the cervix, the lower section of the uterus that opens during labor. Prostaglandins, which can be put into the vagina or taken orally, can be used to treat cervical ripening.

Artificial Membrane Rupture: This involves breaking the amniotic sac that surrounds the infant, which can aid in the stimulation of contractions. This is commonly accomplished with a little plastic hook Inserted via the vaginal canal and into the cervix.

Oxytocin Infusion: Oxytocin is a hormone that promotes uterine contractions. An intravenous (IV) line may be used to administer an oxytocin infusion to help promote labor.

Labor induction can be successful, but it is not without hazards. The procedure is more difficult and time-consuming than natural labor, and it may raise the risk of problems such as fetal distress or the necessity for cesarean delivery. As a result, induction of labor should be performed only when the advantages outweigh the dangers and under thorough medical supervision.

Mode of Distribution

The manner of delivery for diabetic pregnant women is usually selected by the obstetrician depending on several criteria, including the patient's diabetes. The woman's blood sugar management, the growth of the fetus, the presence of any diabetes problems, and the mother and baby's overall health.

Vaginal delivery is generally favored if the mother's blood sugar is well controlled, the fetus is of normal size, and there are no other issues that might need a C-section. A C-section may be suggested to ensure a safe birth if the fetus is big or there are worries about the baby's health.

Women with diabetes should explore their delivery alternatives with their healthcare team and devise a plan that takes their unique requirements and circumstances into account.

Postnatal Care

Postpartum care is the medical treatment and assistance given to a woman after she has given birth. It is a crucial element of maternal health care since it aids in the promotion of recovery, the prevention and management of problems, and the mother's adjustment to her new position as a caretaker.

Postpartum care is especially critical for diabetic women since they are at a higher risk of problems such as postpartum hemorrhage, infection, and blood sugar swings. The healthcare staff will usually give you information on how to self-monitor your blood sugar levels, correct nutrition and water, and physical activity suggestions. They also keep a tight eye on the mother for any signs of problems.

Additionally, the healthcare team may offer breastfeeding advice, contraceptive advice, and emotional support for postpartum sadness or anxiety. It is critical for diabetic women to continue their regular postpartum care to ensure the best possible health results for both the mother and the baby.

Breastfeeding With Diabetes

Breastfeeding has several advantages for both the mother and the baby, and women with diabetes are encouraged to nurse their children. Breastfeeding can aid in the regulation of the baby's blood sugar levels as well as the promotion of healthy growth and development. Breastfeeding can help reduce the mother's risk of acquiring type 2 diabetes and other health issues.

Diabetes patients may need to take extra measures when breastfeeding. Blood sugar levels must be regularly monitored, and insulin or other drugs must be adjusted as needed. To avoid hypoglycemia, women with type 1 diabetes may need to increase their carbohydrate intake while breastfeeding.

It is also critical to continue regular postpartum care to ensure the best possible health results for both the mother and the baby.

Collaborate with healthcare providers to ensure that the baby is getting enough milk and growing normally. Diabetes increases the risk of inadequate milk supply or delayed lactation, and women with diabetes may require additional assistance or measures to ensure successful nursing.

Overall, breastfeeding can be a safe and beneficial choice for mothers with diabetes and their infants with proper monitoring and assistance.

7

Postpartum Care

Blood Sugar Management Following Delivery

Blood sugar levels in women with gestational diabetes normally return to normal within a few days of delivery. However, women with a history of gestational diabetes should continue to be monitored, they should monitor their blood sugar levels after delivery since they are more likely to acquire type 2 diabetes later in life.

Healthcare practitioners may advise frequent blood sugar testing in the immediate postpartum period to ensure that levels remain steady. They may also advise a six- to twelve-week postpartum oral glucose tolerance test (OGTT) to look for evidence of chronic diabetes or impaired glucose tolerance. A good diet and frequent physical activity, for example, can also aid with blood sugar control after birth. Breastfeeding mothers must keep their blood sugar levels steady to ensure an adequate milk supply.

Women who have a history of gestational diabetes should be aware of the signs and symptoms as well: Increased thirst, frequent urination, impaired vision, and exhaustion are among the symptoms of type 2 diabetes. Regular medical check-ups can aid in the early detection and control of type 2 diabetes.

Breastfeeding and Medications

When nursing, it is critical to consider medication safety. Some drugs may pass through breast milk and may harm the infant. Before taking any medicine while nursing, it is critical to contact a healthcare expert regarding its safety. In the case of diabetic drugs, some can be taken safely while breastfeeding, while others are not. Insulin, for example, is typically regarded as safe to take during breastfeeding. However, some oral diabetes drugs, such as metformin, may transfer into breast milk in trace levels, and their use should be avoided. The safety of breastfeeding is unknown. It is critical to discuss any drug and breastfeeding problems with a healthcare provider.

Follow-up Treatment

Follow-up treatment is an important element of controlling diabetes after childbirth. Women with diabetes should see their healthcare practitioner six weeks after delivery for a postpartum checkup. Blood sugar levels will be examined, and the healthcare professional will review the woman's overall health, including any issues related to diabetes during pregnancy, during this visit.

In addition to the postpartum checkup, women with diabetes should continue to monitor their blood sugar levels on a regular basis and maintain a healthy lifestyle that includes a balanced diet and regular physical activity. Women who are pregnant should have their blood sugar levels monitored 6-12 weeks postpartum to confirm that their blood sugar levels have returned to normal. Women with preexisting diabetes will require continued diabetes control after giving birth.

Breastfeeding can also aid in the management of blood sugar levels following delivery. Breastfeeding can help regulate blood sugar levels and improve insulin sensitivity, making it an ideal option to manage diabetes in the postpartum period. Diabetes patients who are breastfeeding should continue to test their blood sugar levels on a regular basis and make any required changes to their diabetes management plan under the supervision of their healthcare professional.

Overall, diabetes must be managed continuously during the postpartum period to avoid complications and preserve the health of both the mother and the infant. Regular monitoring and follow-up care are essential for success. This is the goal.

Options for Contraception

It is critical for diabetic women to consider contraception choices after giving delivery. There are several methods available, and the best way may be determined by personal characteristics such as medical history, lifestyle, and personal preferences. Contraception methods that are regularly utilized include:

Barrier methods, such as condoms and diaphragms, work by physically preventing sperm from accessing the egg.

Hormonal techniques: Hormones are used in these treatments, such as pills, patches, or injectables, to suppress ovulation and/or thicken cervical mucus, preventing sperm from reaching the egg.

Long-acting Reversible Contraception (LARC): LARC treatments, such as the intrauterine device (IUD) or contraceptive implant, enable long-term contraception without requiring daily monitoring.

Sterilization: Surgical procedures such as tubal ligation are available or vasectomy, provide long-term contraception.

Women with diabetes should explore their options with their healthcare professionals because some procedures may be more appropriate than others based on individual health needs and preferences. It's also crucial to think about how the approach, you choose may affect your blood sugar control and any potential drug interactions with diabetic drugs.

8

Long-Term   Health
Consequences

Women with gestational diabetes are more likely to develop type 2 diabetes later in life. As a result, women with a history of gestational diabetes must maintain a healthy lifestyle that includes a nutritious diet, frequent physical activity, and weight management.

The chapter also highlights the significance of frequent health check-ups and blood sugar monitoring. Women who have had gestational diabetes should be evaluated for type 2 diabetes every three years, and more frequently if they have risk factors including obesity or a family history of diabetes, such as excessive blood pressure and cholesterol.

Overall, the chapter emphasizes the need of adopting proactive efforts after pregnancy to avoid or control diabetes and related health issues to ensure long-term health and well-being.

Diabetes Management Following Pregnancy

Diabetes management after pregnancy is critical for long-term health and well-being. Here are some post-pregnancy diabetes control tips:

- To maintain regular blood sugar monitoring and adjust therapy as needed.

- Maintain a nutritious diet rich in fruits, vegetables, whole grains, lean proteins, and healthy fats. Cut down on your intake of processed and high-fat foods.

- Regular physical activity, such as walking or swimming, can help you maintain a healthy weight and control your blood sugar levels.

- Take any medications, including insulin, as directed by your healthcare professional.

- Attend regular check-ups with your doctor to evaluate your blood sugar levels, blood pressure, and other health factors.

- Maintain regular health checks, such as eye checkups and renal function tests.

- Seek the assistance of healthcare experts, diabetes educators, and support groups to help you manage your diabetes and live a healthy lifestyle.

Women with diabetes can effectively manage their illness and lower their risk of long-term health consequences by following these suggestions.

Preparing For a Future Pregnancy

Preparing for future pregnancies is an important factor for diabetic women. A preconception consultation with a healthcare provider is advised to explore any potential hazards and optimize blood sugar control prior to conception.

During this session, the healthcare provider may recommend medication and insulin dose adjustments as well as further tests and monitoring during pregnancy. Concerns regarding potential consequences, including pre-eclampsia and prenatal hypertension, must also be addressed.

Women with diabetes who want to get pregnant should be informed of the increased risk of birth abnormalities and take steps to improve their health before getting pregnant. Quitting smoking, reducing alcohol intake, and maintaining a healthy weight are some examples.

Regular monitoring and follow-up treatment with a healthcare provider during and after pregnancy can also help to ensure the mother and baby's ideal health outcomes.

Considerations for Emotional and Mental Health

Managing emotional and mental health is an important element of post-pregnancy diabetes management. Diabetes management stress can have an emotional impact Postpartum depression, anxiety, or other mental health issues may occur in some women. It is critical to seek assistance and support whenever necessary.

To address emotional and mental health concerns, healthcare providers may send women to mental health experts, support groups, or counseling programs. Furthermore, regular follow-up consultations with healthcare experts can assist monitor mental well-being and make any changes to treatment regimens.

Self-care practices such as regular exercise, proper food, and appropriate rest can also aid in emotional and mental health management. Having a support system in place, such as family and friends, to offer assistance and encouragement during the postpartum period is essential.

Conclusion

Diabetes during pregnancy does not automatically result in death. Women with diabetes can have good pregnancies and give birth to healthy kids with correct management and care. Working closely with healthcare experts, following a nutritious diet, routinely monitoring blood sugar levels, engaging in regular physical activity, and taking any prescribed medications as suggested are all vital. Regular prenatal care, including fetal monitoring, can also aid in the identification and management of potential diabetic issues throughout pregnancy. While women with diabetes may have additional challenges and considerations during pregnancy, with the correct care and management, they can have successful pregnancies and healthy babies.

While controlling diabetes during pregnancy can be difficult, women with diabetes can have good pregnancies and birth healthy babies with adequate care and management.

It is critical to work to properly manage blood sugar levels, work together with a healthcare team, keep regular monitoring and follow-up appointments, and make lifestyle changes. Women with diabetes can boost their chances of a successful pregnancy and ensure long-term health for themselves and their offspring by adopting these precautions.